Love

Handles

A Story of finding love and the weight gain as a result of it

Teka Rose

Love

Handles

A Story of finding love and the weight gain as a result of it

DEDICATION

For My husband and my sons, who have not only put up with me through this health journey, but have walked with me. To my Mother and Poppy, thank you for always being an inspiration and spiritual counselors and helped me to "Put Jesus first". Thank you.

CONTENTS

Chapter One:

Ahh, Love!

So we've all been here before…in love. Such a wonderful, elating feeling to have someone in your life that's not like that last lover; this is it! True love has grabbed hold of you and ran away with your heart. Maybe not, maybe you just really like hanging out with this person, either way the relationship exists. It has already begun for you. You are here. Sexy, single and ready to mingle is such a true statement.

We all start out trying to look our version of our own personal best and do a damn good job of it if we must say so ourselves. You go to your respective watering hole of choice, your library, coffee shop or park on the prowl. Mr. or Mrs. Right is going to get it now. Point is you're maintaining a version of yourself that you feel is presentable to others. Maybe not your main or only goal in life is to find that special someone, but the option is always out there and you're ready for them.

Let's face it; this is no longer the era of the 50's homemaker. You know the plump mom who's always baking and waiting for you to get home from school. It's a new day of Bootylicious, Fergilicious super women who be up in the gym, just a workin' on their fitness. The cast of <u>Oceans Eleven</u> alone is enough to motivate men to push themselves to Metro sexual greatness. Competition is fierce, so staying afloat is quite the daily task that we are more than up to as the party of one we currently are.

But then it happens. You find what you've been looking for in that special someone. You are head over heels and they are perfect. Your eyes meet across a crowded room, you jog past them in the park or they move into your building across the hall. You're interested and hoping for the best, and you're just about to get it. Then, of all the mean, selfish and inconsiderate things to do in the world they do to you; invite you out to dinner. I know it seems great that this has just happened. But little do you know it's only the beginning of a very destructive future. Yes destructive, but we'll get to that later on. Dinner has repeated itself twice this week and not to forget about that nightcap at the coffee shop. Then, it's to the movies next week to see the next big flick of the season. Even something seemingly so innocent as a poetry reading turns into three glasses of wine. Point is, many activities out there that couples partake of are fun, exciting, and oh so full of calories! I know there are many people out there who would disagree, or say just stay active, but truth is unless you both are health nuts, or extreme workout buddies this scenario applies to you…and your spouse.

The end result of your dating actions has yet to rear its ugly head, but read on my friends, it only gets better from here. Me personally, it started out as a single trip to the movies. We dated daily from then on; from him making delicious dinners, to quick stops at fast food joints before we went out, or in for movie night to romantic lunches while visiting the other at work. When it comes to matters of the heart, food happens.

Many of us will get away with maintaining ourselves

below the weight gained radar for years. It's a tricky art for most, but for some it comes natural because you may be naturally slim or slender. So you have eluded the fat demons for quite some time; but they are tricky devils, hence the name demons. They will try and try again to get you, watch your back. We all know the average size of the American woman is a lovely size 14 and blah, blah, blah. I personally feel I look my best at a size 10, but you know, in my adult life I've never been smaller than that so I'm not quite sure how I look with the seemingly obligatory six pack. I digress. My point is if your body is not naturally built to sustain the fast life of love, then the weight will come, no question. A social butterfly such as me is the perfect victim of this life. She loves hanging out with friends, and eating. She attends lavish or maybe even the old school house party, and eating. A night out with the girls, eating and drinking and so it goes. I'm not putting all the blame on the women, but our bodies are more susceptible to the things we put in it.

Love is a beautiful thing, and in the beginning its all that matters at the time, but be weary my friends. That cloud nine feeling will be the end of your once flattering figure if you're not careful.

Chapter Two:

Does this relationship make me look Fat?

It's been a few weeks, months or you even got away with a few years. Things are still great, but you notice those cute outfits don't fit like they used to. Your honey, still in the throes of love thinks the extra pounds are cute or flattering. Maybe so, but you aren't feeling just as convinced that they are that it's okay. Let the yo-yoing begin!

You decide that you want to rid yourself of these few extra pounds and first things first. The decision to do so has been made up in your mind. "I will eat no sweets, less sugar and no junk food!" Such great ideas. You pick up a six pack of the most flavorful diet soda; buy enough cans of tuna to feed a tiny village and rice cakes to get you through the day. Just typing that makes me want a cheeseburger! Don't get me wrong, you have the right idea.

Eating healthier is the start of changing your dietary way of life. Eighty percent of being healthy is nutrition. I'm in no way knocking workouts; we'll just get to that later. You're damn right to want to rid your home of the evil cookies that goes so well with your honey's signature hot chocolate. But, you must pick the right things for yourself that will be a balance of the things you want and of the things you *need*.

I am an avid fan of food and have the ultimate displeasure of being able to picture the looks, taste, and smell of the things I am craving. Then it's so real, I make it manifest. To tell the truth I really am not a junk food eater.

I love my broccoli, fruits and pretty much every vegetable out there. But I do not eat at the right time of day, I skip breakfast often. I am a rice and potato addict, and not to mention, when I do eat beef, I really don't mind the fat on my steak. These are just not good choices. Little tweaks will begin the trend to a better way of feeding myself. Lean cuts of meat, more veggies than anything else on the plate, and of course, portion control. I also never knew that drinking plenty of water can increase your metabolism…increase my metabolism! Without those fad pills that cost $39.99 or more, I can just drink more water to do that? Wow, I've wasted so much money on those damn pills; I could just kick myself…if I could get my leg up there.

This is how a lot of us feel at this stage of our relationship. We dare not reveal to our sweetie how we're feeling though, because they may feel we're being insecure or worse agree with us. What torment, so we continue on, in our own personal secret journey to right this wrong. For some strange reason things aren't working out as planned. You're doing pretty well throughout the day with the plan, skipping meals and whatnot. Maybe even just eating a late dinner with the honey and sharing their dessert.

What we're not realizing is the fact that those missed meals are missed opportunities to gain energy, proteins and nutrients required to keep our bodies going. Those late dinners with the love of your life could be a little earlier and that plate could be a little lighter. A late dinner means an even later dessert…now where do you think your brownie or ice cream is sitting when you kiss them goodnight and lie down? Not to the ab factory my friends, it's going to the bigger ass factory. You could've had so much more of that tuna on a cracker for lunch too. I'm not judging you, actually jus sharing some of my personal story with you.

The focus here, does not need to be how skinny can I get, it needs to be more of a "how healthy am I?" I personally, at this point am not very healthy myself. But this will be a journey for us both. Literally, as I sit here and now I am starting my journey, for the umpteenth time for a healthier me. I would tell you how much I weigh, but that would mean revealing it to my husband of almost ten years, so I'll just let you know how much I've lost at the end of this. Though remember, it's not about the numbers on the scale (although they don't have t be so high) it's about the health your wanting to achieve. The longevity of life, the confidence in yourself for setting goals and not only reaching them but maintaining them. A changing of the tides, in your favor of course. So stop asking if you look fat in those jeans, you know how the hell you look in them. Obviously YOU think you look fat in them, so its time to do something about it. BUY A BIGGER PAIR! Just kidding, unless you need to, we can't have people walking around in the unmentionables now can we? Although your honey may love it; they may think you are the finest thing they've ever seen.

As cute as a couple as you are, you're still an individual, so it's still how you feel about yourself. That being said, let's get cracking!

Chapter Three:

K.I.S.S YOURSELF!

So here it begins. You've made the choice…no wait; you've made the DECLARATION to change your habits and do better for yourself. But where to start?

If you can afford it, visit a nutritionists or trainer that best fits your style of need. We must reiterate style of need because I've encountered several trainers that were awesome at what they do but I awesomely hated their approach to my personal goals and found myself quitting. Dodging their calls, and ignoring their tutelage, only to my own disadvantage. But finding someone who understands nutrition as well as physical needs is important to keep you motivated and can cater to you personally. Not some one size fits all regimens. I now am not able to afford either being a working wife and mother of two and technically considered lower middle class, so we live check to check. So, I'm left to fend for myself and literally become an information sponge. Now I have matched my literal and figurative features…lol.

There is so much information out there on proper nutrition and weight loss it will not be as easy as that. You must do research and stick with the plan that best fits your needs; but keep it simple. Go back to the basics so to speak. Here are a couple of steps to keeping it simple:

K   **Keep to the outer ring of the grocery store**
I   **Identify the good and bad foods in your life**
S   **Stay hydrated!**
S   **Stay active. Even at 20% its super important**

Sounds easy enough right? One would think but there's a reason you should follow this regimen closely, it's not just a reason to pucker up to your honey!

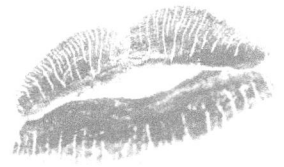

Keeping to the outer ring of the grocer is important because that's where you'll find the basic of good nutrition foods: Meat, Fruits, Vegetables, Diary, breads are all the tools you should need. The inner aisles of grocery stores are jam packed with processed, genetically modified foods and all kinds of junk for quick fix types of lifestyle. Now, if you're a mother like me that is THE go to place for all things children. But why must it be this way? Because little Christian will be such a terror if he doesn't get his juicy juice and chewy snacks? Well tough titty! Because we weren't trained properly in nutrition doesn't mean we have to keep the vicious cycle of misinformation tricking down to our now overweight and or malnutrition offspring. It's also very important that while sticking to the meats, fruits and vegetables to be sure it's organic, locally grown is even better! I only say this because I am now learning more about substances that are put into what seem like trustworthy brands and food that are not healthy for you.

That's the "GRAS FOOD" and it should be avoided at all possible cost. GRAS is the label the FDA has put into select chemicals and ingredients that are "Generally Recognized as Safe". That being said sounds dumber to me every time I hear it. If you were at a restaurant and asked the waiter about today's special and his response was well…it's generally recognized as safe so we're making it! You'd probably stand up and walk out of there. If it a one single ingredient that you cannot safely eat a spoonful of and not die, then it's not safe. PERIOD. And that ingredient was only added to enhance the flavor or size of the food to increase the amount charged if buying by the pound. Or simply so it lives longer on the shelf and doesn't expire.

We have been subjected to the greed of companies for

far too long and horribly misinformed. The information is available to you; you just have to find it. There are currently 373 different chemicals that are on this list that are given the okay to be put into your food, drinks and make-up. I clearly cannot list all the harmful additives here, but it available for you to find. Some may quite surprising, others quite disturbing finds and may feel like a huge undertaking to have to do the research. Ask yourself, am I worth it? Is my family worth it? If you all are, it is a lifestyle change... a big one. But that's why it's a lifestyle and not a get thin quick type deal.

This information helps EVERYONE! We can only benefit from it by educating ourselves and others around us. It will be a process. It helps our young to develop better and healthier habits for themselves that they too can pass down starting a new tradition of health. As you learn this you will want to share the information with your honey! It will get them excited and wanting to learn more as well.

Now you're both learning new things you never knew about food and your relationship can actually benefit from this change! It's something fresh and new that you can experience together. Try out new restaurants with your new food interests in mind. Try new wines and beverages you didn't know were available to you. Gradually as you condition yourself to the new lifestyle, you're figure will be the better for it, and yes, both of you have noticed. That's enough to earn some real kisses!

Identifying the good and bad foods in your life can be done with researching on your own or with the help of a nutritionist. It's a very specific process that will be structured only for you; everyone's needs are different. It will also be a process you conduct throughout your lifestyle change and not just something that will happen in the beginning stages.

As you learn and try new foods, some make be beneficial to your health goals, some may not and some you just may not like whatsoever. There are always alternatives to receiving necessary vitamins and nutrients in certain foods. This is a good time for you and your significant other to shop together, choose foods you both love and foods you may prefer as individuals. Being in love does not mean you always love the same things! Have tastes tests for each other…who knows what it may lead to!

Staying hydrated sounds super easy, but is a little more difficult than one would think if they're not used to drinking the required amounts of water. People in transition will choose to try to slowly "downgrade" from the more harmful drinks; like sugar filled sodas, teas and fruit juices. They tend to want to "drink healthier" products or what they at least think is healthy like, light fruit juices, diet drinks teas and performance type energy drinks.

Most of these you actually need to avoid as well. Many of them tend to contain some of those harmful additives as we mentioned earlier. One main additive to diet drinks is Saccharin; an artificial sugar substitute is commonly made by combining anthranilic acid (used among other things as a corrosive agent for metal) with nitrous acid, sulfur dioxide, chlorine, and ammonia. You read that right, doesn't sound so sweet now does it? It has been linked to a variety of allergic reactions, breathing issues, skin rashes, headaches and bowel control issues such as diarrhea. Not only is that a romance killer, but it's just not sexy! So steer clear of those additives.

The performance enhancers are a mix; some are good some are just loaded with sugar. Read your labels thoroughly. The few that are good should be consumed only for pre or post workouts and should not be in any way a replacement for the amount of water you need daily. Believe it or not the saying "drink 8 cups of water a day" does not apply. The amount of water you both need, will vary based on your weight. Be sure you check to see how much is recommended for you, it should be an easy find online or by consulting with your physician. You may also want to research the benefits of water other than tap or bottled water, because some may contain additives based on the manufacturer, and again I urge you to read your labels and do your research!

Staying active should be a given. A rolling stone gathers no moss; well a person in motion gains no fat…well, less fat. You get the point! Although eighty percent of your health is nutrition, that remaining twenty percent is very important as my spouse and I have learned.

Even with the strictest of diets, you should still be as active as possible for your heart health, bone and joint health and general well-being. If you're anything like most people, time is a critical factor for you. Maybe you have no time in the mornings before work or in the evening after. It's possible you're pooped from an exhausting day. But exercise should be like that pair of jeans you are longing to fit back into; you gotta get in where you fit in. If you don't make the time, you won't be fitting into those jeans anytime soon. This being said, you can hear all the clichés in the world, they're all applicable to what you want, but none help with the time factor, or motivation for that matter. So what's a person to do?

You must make a plan that works best for you and stick with it! Maybe you and your honey can schedule something together. This works for some couples because it not only gives you time together, but it helps to give you both a chance to be each other's coach, companion and support system. You can challenge each other to reach a specific goal, you can compete with one another for weight or inches lost or you can simply motivate each other during your workout. Be it at the gym or at your home there are many different options you can choose that best suit you as to what will make it obtainable.

If your schedules do not permit a tandem workout, then you can still plan something together on paper to be executed separately. If you choose this route; plan to meet up to discuss the goals you set, your daily or weekly progress made or even any falters in the planning. Falters happen. That doesn't mean revert to eating poorly and giving up. Even if it's a falter in meals or workouts, let that be your only one…I say this because too often we'll falter via food or missing a workout and then justify the rest of the day's missteps because of that one. You must get out of that pattern!

If you ate a doughnut at work, that does not mean go ahead with the cheeseburger and fries for lunch; it simply means you had a doughnut. It was delicious and maybe not a part of your meal plan, but it happened. Continue with your meal plan as it was intended and complete your workout. That's it. Don't beat yourself up over that choice. Whatever you do, don't try to justify it either, it's those justifications that get us because they tend to multiply and before you know it have derailed all of your goals.

If working with your partner is not an option at all, then make your plans for yourself and communicate any needs to them. Those needs could be simply a mental support system or asking them not to bring certain foods into the home. This may be easier said than done. Not every couple will be on the same page as far as fitness and health goals. If this is the case for you, you'll have to have extra discipline and willpower.

There may be plenty of temptations around to demotivate you. That can include the temptation not to work out because your honey is on the couch or in the bed watching a good movie. Resist that urge to cuddle up if you have a workout that needs to be done. Who knows, that determination may motivate them to join in! As always, do the research for yourself to see what works best for you and your body type. Maybe hitting the gym isn't for you. You may prefer home workouts. If that isn't the case for you, there are so many activities and classes that you can do to get your blood pumping and burn calories. Walking, Dancing, Yoga, Martial Arts or even joining a team sport are a few different options. A lot of cities have team sports you can join solo or as a couple. Check online for the ones that may be offered near you.

If you have children, go outdoors and play a game of Basketball or dodge ball. You'll have fun spending time with your kids as well as work up a great sweat! This may not be done daily, so you will still need to incorporate other activities for the remainder of the week. But this may help to break up your workouts so they don't feel like an obligation. If it feels like an obligation, its eventually going to feel like a burden, leading to it more likely being something you don't want to stick with.

Make it fun! Just keep moving as much as possible so you can enjoy those date nights out at the restaurant and don't have to feel guilt. The sole purpose is to stay active daily. You can schedule work out for specific days and follow through with them. But even in your typical day to day, do things different to keep active. Take the stairs instead of the elevator, park at the far end of a parking lot and walk to the store…if possible leave the car home and actually WALK to the store! Go out dancing sans the drinks, you'd be amazed at how many calories you can burn dancing. Stay in with your sweetie and dance together that may even lead to more calories burned. There are many things you can do to remain active at home, just get creative and get moving.

Chapter Four

Make It Official

Well you've done so incredibly well thus far, great job! Your diet and exercise have been maintained like never before, you're working out and feeling great and both you and your beau have noticed the amazing changes. Now what? Now is the time to decide to make it official and keep with your regime that has helped you come this far. It has to be a lifestyle change, not a diet. The efforts you've made wasn't just to fit into a dress or look good for the summer…you always want that triumph over the battle of the bulge.

The only way to achieve that is to live your life to be a conscious, healthier you! The choices you make every day will directly affect your figure, your attitude and your overall general health. So let them be good ones. Consistent with all of the wonderful choices you have made thus far.

Your health is the most important thing in your life next to your spouse and their health and well-being. So if you love one another, act like it and love them to be a healthier them. It's been said that it takes thirty days of doing something consistently for it to become a habit. So if you've been on track for at least that long, then you should be used to your routine by now. If not, stick with it! The payoff will come sooner than you think.

I have been a victim of failed immediate results. In a

society of instant gratification, it's no wonder. Someone can eat poorly, never exercise have their bodies show that slothfulness and go into a plastic surgeon and have it all taken away. But if you think about it, they are simply starting over again because they have not developed the good habits that come with maintaining yourself. They have only placed a band aid over a gaping wound. It's bound to get infected. That's exactly what a quick fix does, makes it okay for a short period, but in the end becomes more of a hassle for not taking the time to fix it properly. I wanted to be skinny, not skinny, drop dead gorgeous shapely. I'm not there yet, but have learned so much more about my body and what it needed to be healthy. So I have made serious strides…leaps and bounds and my husband has surely taken notice!

So that's your next step in this journey of amazing, positive health transformation. TAKE NOTICE! Time will surely show all your efforts and hard work. Not only on your physical appearance outside, but your physical well-being on the inside will show everyone the difference. Your body can function at its best levels when it is properly nourished. Your skins glows, your mind is clear and free of clutter and all five of your senses are alive!

Take that leap of faith and make the commitment to yourself. Make the decision to love yourself so much that you will do anything to keep yourself happy. Seek peace and contentment within yourself, and that glow will shine for miles around. Everyone will notice the change. Some may love it, so may not. But they're all thinking the same thing…you've got it going on! Those types of energy can be contagious and make you a magnet. People want to be around genuinely healthy, happy people.

So let them gravitate to you and share the knowledge you've learned and taught yourself. It will only further benefit our society and our culture. How great would this world be if everyone was happy and content with themselves? It sounds like it may be on too large a scale to achieve, but it only takes a spark to start a raging wildfire! If you don't believe that then the diet industry wouldn't be a multi-billion dollar industry. People generally want to look good, but imagine if all of those people felt as good as they looked? Just from a few, simple steps. Something that is well within our reach could change and affect so much!

While you're on this journey, let love be your guide. Your love for yourself, your significant other and friends and family help you. It should all be motivation to stay on track. Your spouse may be on the journey to healthier living with you which is even better. Utilize this time to learn just how far your love can go and grow.

Chapter Five

Don't Fear Change

Both you and your honey have made significant life changes. You've tried new foods, new routines and have probably had many "news" over the past couple of months. That's a great thing! By making the commitment to improve your health you've made many changes already, so why do I say to not fear it? I say this simply because there are going to be even more "new" things that you can discover. I'd like you to explore other life options that may in the long run be a great benefit to your new lifestyle.

Food

You've by now done your research, so you're well aware of some of the health benefits and hindrances certain foods could have. So you may have reduced your portions, or added new foods into your diet. This is a great time to explore new things. Try independent Natural and specialty food stores that promote organic, healthy living. They are usually smaller than your typical grocer, but have a more personable feel.

With that comes the opportunity to learn more about what you ingest and can ask questions of the benefits of the foods they have to offer. Some even support your local farmers and you can buy food if not directly from your town, you can bet its close! Certain people may say those stores are too expensive, but if you're the smart savvy shopper I know you are then finding great deals won't be hard for you. Not to mention, supply and demand, the greater the demand, the better deals or concessions can be made to you as a consumer if the market is competitive.

I'm not suggesting you have to become a Vegetarian or Vegan, a lot of these stores sell fresh organic meat as well. You'll learn the benefits of what you eat as you go. In the meantime, don't knock the idea though; it's a very healthy and rewarding lifestyle too. So if the thought of abandoning your favorite grocery store terrifies you, start small. Buy only small items here and there at first, get comfortable with your surroundings and ask questions. Lots of them, you'll be happy you did!

Nutrition

Yes, food is a vast part of your nutrition, but you must be aware of exactly what nutrients your body is getting or not getting. If you decided to forgo meat for instance, you will need to supplement those lost vitamins and nutrients that come with consuming meat. You may want to discuss with your physician or nutritionist what options are available to you so your body gets what it needs to function.

Some people choose supplements; others prefer not to have to take pills. So if you have deleted meat from your existence you have alternate foods that will give you what you need. Nuts, Seeds, Spinach, Quinoa, Soy, beans and select dairy products just to name a few. Most of these may already be in your diet. Point is, simply because you've chosen to go without certain meal doesn't mean you have to starve your body of the important nutrients it needs. So read up, and educate yourself on what will work best for you at home. Experiment in the kitchen together!

Exercise

Your new workout routine has done wonders for you and you love the feeling you get when you've accomplished yet another workout. Be careful not to become complacent in your routine. It can become a drag to do after a while if you don't switch it up. If you decided to join a gym for instance and have been only focusing on cardio and love your results, you may want to stick to only cardio.

That's not an issue, but your body is built to adapt to its conditions. So if you're doing the same cardio routine day in and day out, it won't be a challenge for your body much longer. You won't see the amazing results you once were. This is where you must switch it up! Maybe throw in some weight training into your routine. Join a class that may be offered at your gym, like Zumba, or a belly dancing. Its fun and you can burn a lot of calories doing it. If you chose a home workout regimen, do the same.

Perhaps decide to walk outside instead of staying in on equipment or doing that same workout DVD. If your experience is anything like mine was, I actually own more than twenty fitness DVD's! All a result of failed attempts at getting fit quick schemes. I'm in no way knocking the DVD's themselves, but when I didn't see the instant results I was looking for after a few days, I gave up on them. So they sat around my home for years, some waiting to be watched once.

Their dream came true and that was actually the

beginning of my journey to health. When I did decide to change my life, I couldn't afford to rejoin my gym, so I wrote out a plan and included every one of those orphaned workout DVD's. I did one DVD consistently for six days, and rested on the seventh. The next week, I started a new one. That truly challenged my body because of the plethora of different exercises I was putting myself through. I also decided to walk in my neighborhood every evening after dinner and to my surprise enjoyed it very much.

Soon, my husband started to join me and we used it as a time to talk about any and everything we wanted. We both looked forward to that added privacy away from our kids. If there is something you've always wanted to try, get out and DO IT. You have nothing to lose.

There are tons of options on healthy activities to keep you moving and on the right track. But for lists sake, I'll name a few: Swimming, hiking, biking, dancing, white water rafting, boot camps, sports teams, Yoga, running and oh so many more! It's your choice; you just have to make it.

Spirituality

You may not be a spiritual person. I strongly am, I believe that God has blessed me with all that I am and all that I have. I also believe in a having a deep and centered connection with your soul.

What I mean by that is you may pray daily or you may read spiritual guides often, but sometimes you simply need to sit down and connect with yourself…your soul. I am still on my own spiritual journey so I'll keep my personal opinions short on this matter. I believe it's very important we each seek out our own understanding of how to live our lives.

Meditation has helped me to ground myself and center my thoughts. It's also a time I used to pray and show my thankfulness for all that I have and all I have been able to accomplish in my personal journey. It's refreshing and makes me feel good as a whole. This is why I was moved to include this for you.

I have learned meditation poses in doing yoga and I'll add my own prayers. I have studied other cultures practices and have picked out things I like most about them and now included mantras, chants and focusing on my chakras as well. I not only feel more centered within myself, but I also feel a certain connection with the earth.

Now don't go getting all "she's lost it" on me, what I mean is that when I'm grounded I feel a connection with all that surrounds me and I become more aware of not only myself, but of all things. I appreciate the elements more, I respect their strength and power, I know where they came from and Who created them, and I am more thankful for these things that I was oblivious to prior to meditation. I must reiterate, that this is not something that you may like or that I am pushing on you, but if you try it, you may like it. All I ask is that you make the decision to EXPLORE other things to improve your quality of life. Study cultures other than your own; you may learn some very valuable information and practices.

Once your body is cleansed and free of all the harmful things that it once was used to, your mind will clear and you may be directed to spiritual enlightenment of your own accord. It's a practice that is nice to have and will also add balance to your life.

Chapter Six

Today's THE Day!

After 14 years of being all "cupcaked" up as my husband would say, those cupcakes have taken their sugary toll on my physique. Throw in a couple of kids, a highly active social life filled with almost any drink you can order from the bar and a few hundred family dinners, get-togethers and cookouts and you've got a woman determined. Determined to shed more than a few unwanted pounds and a spouse to match.

We've decided the best strategy to embark on this journey of leading healthy lives is to attack it together. We gained them together and will work on losing them together, as one. Utilizing his willpower and he my determination to learn all things healthy, we are team up with health experts in our area and beginning the rest of our lives together as a healthy, happy couple. You can do the same with your spouse. Maybe they're not on board at first, mine wasn't either. But they will get on board with you once they witness your dedication for change and growth. Any self-respecting relationship needs this constantly, and it's inevitable.

So you've done everything as planned and got some things that wasn't quite part of the vision. You found love, and it's been great! But pounds found you, and that wasn't so great. Then you decided to K.I.S.S yourself and begin your journey to change. Your shopping habits have been altered and you look at food with a different eye. Carefully considering calories, fats and your portions; you've explored alternative eating options and have visited a few famers markets and natural food stores.

You have made it official in your mind and have begun to learn through trial and error what health options work and what exercise regimens you like and dislike. Maybe you've discovered meditation and all of the stress relieving benefits it has brought. You didn't fear the changes you've made and have embraced the idea of you being a healthier, happier you! Congratulations! Maybe this book has been a guide through the journey you've already begun, or maybe it will serve as the motivation you needed to begin your healthy transformation. Either way, you've opened yourself up to change and if you haven't already started your endeavor, then today is the day.

Grab your best gear, because you want to look good, while you're on a journey to look and feel better! And yes, it does make a difference…you know the term "walk the walk"? Well go get healthy and look like you want to do it! Get your support system lined up, so that you have everyone in your corner and make the changes you've been wanting to make in your life!

As for me and my spouse, we will continue to live in God's word and His will be done, we will grow in our journey together and help others along the way. Our strength and endurance has and will continue to be tested daily, just like yours will, so we will push through together!

Love

Handles

A Story of finding love and the weight gain as a result of it

The next book in the series will follow us in our journey to change our lives and will hopefully become a tool in helping you to begin to change yours! Stay Strong, stay motivated and stay together in love, life and happiness!

ABOUT THE AUTHOR

Teka Rose is a loving wife and mother who resides in Charlotte, North Carolina. Born in Omaha, Nebraska, Teka moved to Charlotte in 1990 with family. Her Passion for Music, Arts and Entertainment helped guide her into a deep love for writing and expression. Motivated purely by love (and the weight gain that came with it), she redirected her lifestyle and shifted her focus to healthy living. Still a lover of all things Music, Arts & Entertainment, Teka has captured the best of both worlds in her Love handles series, and gives her readers a chance to motivate and do the same.

www.ingramcontent.com/pod-product-compliance
Lightning Source LLC
Chambersburg PA
CBHW070938290526
45795CB00003B/1068